ISBN 978-88-6332-053-4

Gabriella Franceschini

JUST A SKIN MATTER

"The year of the cancer" ...

but my sign is Libra!

Translation by Laura Marrocco

Revision by Carmen Fiengo

Edizioni Miele

Acknowledgements

To my family for their endless love.
To Mariateresa Fiumanò for trusting me.
To Francesca Frighi for her patient and
precious technical collaboration.
To Adriana for giving me both good advice
and support, during my delirious states of mind.
To all my irreplaceable "*Adventure Woman*" friends
for the affection, courage and solidarity they
showed me. I love you.
To all the people who is able to understand
"The inner meaning of things", and who believed
in me, even after reading this book.

PREFACE

By Mariateresa Fiumanò

When the "tumor event" affects or interrupts the more or less peaceful course of human existence, above all at young age, it leaves you astonished, amazed that something bad "that usually only happens to other people"has occurred to you, to the body you thought was quite incorruptible and immortal.

A cancer patient very often retires hermetically into his own shell and shut himself away from the world so that he can feel protected by his inner world, but he does not realize that, on the contrary, it can only further increase his suffering. But, fortunately, not everybody reacts in the same way...

This is the story of Gabriella, narrated in the first person, who after a breast cancer diagnosis and surgery, also received radiation therapy.

This is not a sad story about illness, but an optimistic progress leading towards the future.

This is a tale of a brave woman who every day mounts her bicycle and goes, most of the times by herself, to Hospital to receive her increasing range of radiations.

The blue waiting room, that varies its nuances and shades according to the weather and her mood, that for some people, only represents the last chance, for her it is just a hallway to recovery. Here she looks around , commits to her memory and puts into writing an unforgettable testimony of her waiting time, the hopes of a person who, despite her loneliness and deep melancholy, is always ready to donate a bit of herself, her best, to the others. Her cheerfulness and easy going nature is very contagious for her "Adventure Friends", medical attendants, technicians and also the surliest doctors whom, at the end, she succeed to grab a joke from. And now Gabriella is right here, opposite me, with her scar on her brown skin that protected her from the devastating effects of radiations, with her big smile and her book which must and can succeed in giving people hope for the future…

Mariateresa Fiumanò,
a doctor and a friend…

To my mother,
my muse.

To Biri
my muse too.

To the "Dragonfly"...
my unconscious source of inspiration.

1. "The Blue Room"

Everything is blue here.

The walls, the floor, the chairs, even the radiators are blue…and the wait is also blue.

I am sitting here, just waiting for my turn.

This is my first time or rather, this is my first "treatment", as they call it here. I have already done the treatment evaluation, the virtual simulation, the localization of the volume and the tattoo; or better they have drawn three tattoos on my skin, like the brand on cows, on three different areas of my body: the first one under my right armpit, the second one under my left armpit and the third one right at the center of my chest.

I do not want people to compare me to those "yobs" who, back in the past years, used to get "mafia symbols" tattoos on their chest. How dreadful!

Next to me there is my Mother, quite unperturbed and omnipresent. I look at her who, as she pretends to be indifferent, is making crossword puzzles. She inspires me with tenderness, with her sad but proud gaze, being the strong and courageous woman that she is, tender but stubborn as well.

Since the day of my surgery, during these last few months, she has never left me alone. I could have overcome these hurdles and dealt with this bad situation without my mother's support, since I inherited my courage from her, but…it would not have been the same without her.

Mom is always mom!

Her love is unconditional and boundless, like dogs' love, but this is a compliment.

While, I am carelessly leafing through a magazine, I observe my mother's face: she has got wrinkles on her forehead and her face looks tired… I made her look ten years older!

I feel responsible for this but it is not my fault, it is nobody's fault, it is only destiny, the strength tests of life, I know, but I feel responsible anyway.

My mother left Sicily, her daughter (my sister), her two nieces and a three-months old grandniece, just to stay here with me.

I am blessed to have her.

My father stayed at home, drawing him aside because these places are not for him, as he gets scared just looking at a needle.

He… cool and rational, methodical and unapproachable, friendly but also distant, he that can do nothing without my mother.

He is a person who pays taxes one month before the regular due date, fills up his car with gas when the tank is still half-full, "just in case", decelerates his velocity also when the traffic signal is green, since "Who knows? The light could suddenly turn yellow", that can't remember a road that he already covered for hundreds of times and that, above all, is not even able of hugging his daughters. I have no memories of my father ever giving me a hug.

I am absorbed in my own thoughts when the silence is broken by a technician's voice who, looking at my mother, says: "Madam, it is your turn". Everyone always gets this wrong, but my mother and I have become accustomed to this, so we look at each other and smile.

Then he adds: "Come in the Room, take off your necklace, both your t-shirt and bra, then lay down here.

I will come back immediately". Endless minutes.

I look around, even here everything is blue and white.

The "machine", or better "the Medical Linear Accelerator", as they call it, is beyond me. I feel like being at a Solarium.

Three technicians come back and turn around me confusingly saying "Lift up your arms and hold on tight here, don't move at all by any means."

The doctor, a woman, says "Pay attention, you have got a medial scar" … Mumble, mumble!

After activating the medical instruments, she runs away, with the three men, to protect herself.

Just a few minutes of endless thoughts.

After that, "No sun for the entire summer" the doctor warns me.

Gulp, gasp, sgrunt! I love sunbathing!

But…..too many radiations are not good.

2. "What a pity"…

This time the waiting room looks sadder and more blue then ever… maybe the light is different today… I came here by myself with my bike. After my period of convalescence I need to move a bit.

I love to ride my bike, so I also take advantage of this wonderful spring morning!

But… what a pity my "Dragonfly" is not here with me.

There are four women opposite me, all of them over sixty years old… so I think "Wow, I am the youngest one".

I look at them with discretion and I try to imagine their pain, I wonder where their "disease" is… Some of them are with their husbands or their sons and someone is by herself, like me. But I feel calm and quite relaxed. I keep myself company.

What a pity, my friends are not here with me.

Friends, yes… These unknown ones… I don't remember where, but once I read that "Real friends are those rare people who ask how we are and then even wait to hear the answer".

How true!

I even told my friend Rox, 3 months after my surgery and their silence: "Hey, *Cunnuta* ca sì"![1], since she is Sicilian like me,

"Why have you disappeared? I am not contagious at all"!

[1] That is: "*Cunnuta,* here you are". *Cunnuta* is used in Sicilian dialect to mean *cuckquean*, that is the English female equivalent of cuckold and it alludes to "wearing the horns", or rather to husband's infidelity.

Giggles, promises and silence that still lasts.

I don't know but… this situation has taken me back to when I was nine and at school, nobody wanted to sit in the desk with me because I was dark skinned and I came from Africa. I belonged to one of the many families of Italian refugees, forced to repatriate from Libya (I still remember the soldiers with machine-guns under my house and the curfew), to a Country, Italy, that was not ready to receive us yet and so was not our Country.

Anyway it was my mother's decision: "I want to go to Rome, the heart of Italy, so we can be halfway between our relatives from the North and the South of the Country. And then, in Rome there is the sea and, above all, the sun!" She, always so practical and ingenious at the same time.

Since then, I have always been looking for my own place in the world.

Meanwhile, before coming back home, I decide to go to the Arab greengrocer as I want to buy a lot of fruit and vegetables, as they are very good for you.

Salam, Schukràn.

3. "Under the Sun of Rome"

"Only for this Saturday, then we shall start again from Monday to Friday."
They explain me that I can't receive only two treatments and then stop for the weekend.
So, I take up my dear old bike (I should change it, as its wheels are so heavy, but I am very fond of it) and, under a Sun that regenerates, I cover the way that leads me to the Blue Room.
There are not many people since it is Saturday. Two men, with a resigned expression on their face, are probably waiting for their wives. One of them sometimes looks out the window to check and smiles at his little dog that he was forced to tie to a bench outside in the yard.
Whenever the little dog sees him, wags his tail with great happiness.
"Dogs…they are all the same" I think smiling, "whenever you leave them only for a moment, they are pretty sure you have abandoned them forever"… but how grateful they are "just" for a smile.
Everyday a different technician and doctor, but the process is always the same: shirt, bra, "lay down here and don't move, please", they tell me every time.
But I'm absolutely still!
Sometimes I even hold my breath not to move.
The technician on duty today is a bit sour and unfriendly, but I don't care at all.
I am only thinking about having an enjoyable ride as soon as I can go away… under the Sun of Rome.

And... right under the Sun my mobile phone rings... Just a look at the display saying "Mum house", she wants to know how I am and invites me for lunch: "come, mummy's heart, I've prepared a fish dish that is great for your health."

With a big smile on my face, I get on my bike and cycle very fast to her house, searching for nourishment, above all, for my soul.

4. "Whenever I am alone, I break down and cry"

I am quite nervous.

My mother is giving big sighs. It never happened before, or at least I had never seen her doing it. Room B is busy, "Come on baby, I'll take you to a beautiful place". I mechanically follow the technician on duty, who is much nicer than the last one.

He is more talkative, gives me lots of good advice, he is joyful and, as he knows that I am employed in the "Justice System", asks me the name of a talented lawyer. "In a bit you must have a blood test done, as you know, it is very important to control white blood cells"...

"From the tenth treatment on, you will feel a bit drowsy and quite tired, but don't worry, it is normal" ...

Ok.

"You must eat some more since you are very thin"...

Ok.

So he says goodbye with a great smile on his face and goes away with a proud gait. "I wonder why he is laughing... maybe, after so many years of this job, he himself, is a little bit irradiated as well."

My mother is waiting for me in the Blue Room, which today is a bit more blue. My mood, instead, is blue, or rather "dark blue".

We have gone to the Local Health Authority, the INPS office (National Institute of Social Insurance), the Polyclinic, then to the Bank, the personnel department, lots of requests, application forms, revocations, parking, going up and down all day long (this situation reminds me of a scene in a Carlo Verdone's film "*Lift up granny's legs, and then take down granny's legs*")…

Bureaucracy will kill me but... thank goodness I have the disabled parking permit!

I feel very tired today, and it's not even my tenth one, and quite intolerant today. I blamed my mother just for a trivial reason, but immediately afterwards I regretted.

Sometimes when I realize that am treating her very badly, when alone, I break down and cry…Sometimes, on the other hand, I hug her tightly and give lots of kisses on her head, (my mom is quite short indeed) and say "Sorry, Sorry, I love you mommy"…

but then she moves away, pretending to be offended, and sometimes, when she is silent, is really deeply hurt.

I love my sister, even if we are so different but... now I don't have the energy to talk about it.

I log on Windows Messenger…

11: 27 a.m.: "Hi Gabry, are you there?"

Nothing else.

Are these dewdrops too early evaporated?

5. "Behind my silence"

The Sun is shining, it is very hot, so...I can be short-sleeved! It's wonderful!

No bike today. More bureaucracy turnarounds, to INPS again: "Sorry Miss, there's no cheque for you... as you exceed three hundred euro the annual income"... obviously, I thought!

Then mum insists "Come home for lunch, I have prepared the Couscous that you love so much" (sometimes our African origins resurface)... But how can I refuse such a delicious proposal of love?

Only a couple opposite me, probably husband and wife, as they seem to be intimate or maybe they are "adventure companions".

She makes me feel a sense of tenderness with her silver short hair, too short indeed.

A medical attendant pops in the blue room and asks me: "Did you take someone here?"

"No, I am alone" I reply, "I'm just waiting for my turn".

Then I see a nun going out from that "Room" and... I don't know why but... I am quite astonished and find it weird.

I was pretty sure that they were "immunized" of these problems.

We are all God's children, and everyone is loved in the same way, apart from our clothes but... it's a shame that not everyone is equal before the law!

This morning, I decide to send it a message, as ten days

went by since the last time I have heard from it, "I'm around, overwhelmed by bureaucracy, and what about you my "Dragonfly"… did you fly away?"

Absolute silence.

After more than an hour, whereas minutes seem to be centuries, I try, stubbornly, on its second cell number:

"Don't you receive my text messages?… or rather you get them but, because of your own reasons (maybe you are afraid?) you have decided not to reply or… mumble mumble... I don't know…

This time it sends me a reply.

"Gabry, sorry… I have a problem at the office, here I am… see you later, kiss" .

The new technician is quite "plump", with grey hair, beard and wearing glasses, but kind as well. He talks about the weather, "It's too hot to be early spring but, you can't trust April's sun, since you can catch a cold like this".

"He is right", I think. We do not have mid-seasons any-more.

Then he goes on talking while he measures me:

"Lift up your arms, you hang on this, don't move. Ok, perfect!"

I feel almost satisfied.

Before withdrawing in the safety room, he tells me that the next day he has to go to the dentist's, "Phew", he exclaims "There's nothing worse than going to the den-tist's", while the Linear Accelerator rises over me.

"A dark moment in my life…that's the reason of my silence… Kiss".

I turn off my computer then go and take a shower.

6. "We...Southern Women"

I like writing, as it makes me feel good, a bit like reading and listening to music as well.

The Responsible Radiotherapist is a woman. She often smiles, is kind and always greets me. I was not accustomed to this.

The habit, widespread among almost all the doctors, is to talk to you in a hurry, while rushing along the corridors and answering with annoyance to your questions full of hope.

None of them looks into your eyes anymore, and kindness is only an optional. Quite often we are just numbers for them.

The Room B is nearly empty but noisy, I don't know why. Even today my daily routine... early rising, hospital, check-up and colposcopy (now I can understand why it is called in this way, since "colpo" means "blow" in Italian). "Everything is OK, so, come back in a couple of months."

I like to sit here, the last blue chair on the left, near the table and the big window, which enables me to look at the beautiful well-kept garden outside there (strange, in such an ancient hospital), and trees, each one in a different shade of green. I take a deep breath, it is through smells and colors, first of all, that you perceive Spring.

Then "*Ciccillo*", appears at the door... the funny technician who asked me about a talented lawyer. With a great smile he says to me "In a bit it's your turn" and then winks at me.

Ok!

Can we remove our emotions, or decide to deny them? Is this possible? I never succeeded in doing this…

Opposite me there are two women, one of them with very black long hair, the other one with short cropped hair. I can imagine who is accompanying the other one. They are probably friends.

I can hear them chatting and sometimes also laughing.

"They are so tender" I think, whenever I look up they smile at me. I don't know why, but I feel like smoking a cigarette. I desist.

I came here by bicycle so, I might be breathless later.

Ciccillo gave me my coordinates: "84-89-104"… I could bet on them on a lottery, and I could play 10 and 4 and bet on a set of four winning numbers... Uhm!

While going back home, I stop just to eat a banana... it is all potassium, and it is good for your health.

Absolute silence in the house.

My flatmate, "the violinist", has left, she is at Sanremo, but, this time, not for the famous "Italian song's Festival", now she is there for a television broadcast. She is a very good musician, but a little less managing her private life, but I think it is the problem of all musicians and artists as well. But I love her.

We met about six years ago, she had just come from her homeland, Apulia, in the South of the Country, right here in the Capital, the "heart of Italy" Rome, for achieving her dream, her great passion for music. And I must admit that she fully succeeded at it.

We have loved each other since the beginning.

We "Southern Women", recognize one another, we "feel" one another, we are very similar, her and I. Same metabolism, same figure, same star "Libra", with all the particular feelings connected with it.

Anyway, we are also very different in many other respects but, all the same, we balance each other out.

"I realize how difficult can be to understand my silence... when I'm down I close myself into a shell... as I just need to stay like this... but please, don't be hurt, it is only a dark moment. Kiss" .

Ok.

7. "Seven"

Today it is the seventh!

7... it is an important number for me and quite recurring too.

You know, one of those numbers that always follow you, in every life situation and you see them everywhere, also in a cleft... and anyway, seven equals G, the initial of my first name!

Once I named my cat Seven.

That cat was really unique, it used to like so much diving into the bath-tub whenever I was having a bath, but...didn't cats hate water? And then, he would only cross the street on zebra crossings... I know it seems quite crazy but it is true. We use to look at it from the terrace, it was so cautious, one pad along the other, before crossing the road.

And right on zebra crossings... one day... I found it... a life passed away!

I love animals.

I love them, often more than mankind.

This is what a single woman usually thinks, I know, but it's the truth. Anyway among other animals I love dogs because they love you unconditionally, like only a mother can do.

Today the Blue Room is empty.

Maybe I am the first one… or the last one!

Along the journey to get here, I stopped to chat with my former brother-in-law who has a real estate agency right on the street that I cover every day by my bike. Today I saw him smoking outside so, I decided to have an old chat.

He is a funny and witty man always kind with me and, thirteen years after the separation from my sister, (he has abandoned a wife only thirty-years old and two little daughters to chase a love-dream with a twenty-years old woman), our relation has improved. I don't have any grudge towards him for the great suffering he had given my family, "Y*outh mistakes*" he says, and I am pretty sure he is sincere.

I am always his little sister-in-law even if I am older than my sister.

To be in one's 40's ... Time goes by so fast, and she's already a grandmother! The daughter of my niece… It is really so strange…Life goes on implacably.

There is the "plum" one, it's his shift but, he is quiet today, essential, a bit like me.

Why, when you're lying down to watch a ceiling, even just for a few minutes, is your mind so overflowed by thousands of thoughts? They are really thousands, I can't go after them.

The thoughts fly and then come back to you, like a boomerang.

Whenever I meet Tony, inevitably I think of my younger sister, Viviana. It has been three years now, since she moved to Sicily (another important step of our origins), to follow her romantic "love dream" as well. She fell in

love with a Sicilian man, although…
she has always been in love with him, since she was a little girl, when my boyfriend was his twinbrother.
So many promises but never kept.
She moved to Sicily with him and her baby (well… she is sixteen and already taller than 1,70 mt.). Now they live on the beautiful hills of Catania, in a sea view villa, immersed in the green, surrounded by volcanic rocks.
My sister makes me feel a sense of tenderness, she has always made me feel anger and tenderness... but, there is trouble in store for anyone who touches her! As a child she was a pain in the neck, annoying and quite snoopy, like most of younger sisters too…
obviously I am talking as the older one!

"The black sheep", "Who did not get married" like my Sicilian relatives would say about me, "But she is so nice, there is nothing wrong with her!"

8. "The Blowfly and the Dragonfly"

There is a new doctor today. He is very tall and with a heartfelt look. He pops in, observes me quite questioning, and asks: "What's your name?"

There is only a man, standing in front of me, who is probably waiting for his "sweetheart", I can see… he is worried about, moves backwards and forwards… maybe it is their first time. On his head he wears a cap, perfect Sicilian style, he has a gloomy face and wrinkled brow but, as soon as he sees her, suddenly a tender and caring expression appears on his face.

"I am 1,91 mt tall", the Radiotherapist exclaims and then he hastens to add "But all the same, the most important thing is that final 1!"

Duh… "I haven't got a clue!" I think… while he moves around me "Well, hold on tight, good, but… you are very tall!"…

what?… mumble, mumble… meeeeeee?

This is the first time that someone says this to me… I am only 1,64 mt tall but… probably when I lay down, I seem quite taller or maybe the women before my turn were really short indeed.

"Perfect… now you are balanced, well… I am a little bit fussy, as I am from Bergamo"… I didn't know that people from Bergamo were picky.

There is always something new to learn, everywhere.

A fly, or rather a blowfly, diverts the flight of my thoughts.

I see it as soon as the doctor locks himself up in his den,

obviously after warning me in the usual way:

"don't move by any means!"… no way… I follow the blowfly with my eyes (the only organ allowed to move), it runs hither and thither on the ceiling, then disappears...

I breathe a sigh of relief, quite slightly, when… all of a sudden I see it appear once again, a few inches from my face…

Gulp!… my whole body stiffens and I begin to pray:

"don't settle on me… don't settle on me"…

I never thought of having to beg a blowfly!

And finally it does not rely on me.

Who knows how long it has been there, as it flies like crazy and seems to have gone nuts indeed, "maybe the radiation", I think.

What a damn for it to have "taken" on that day right the window of the Blue Room!

I read the first chapter to Tony.

"Go on, please" he says right giving me a boost, "I like the way you write, everything seems quite natural"… may be.

I decide to join the gym, the Official Selection process for "*Adventurewoman*" is just around the corner and if I want to join it I must be in shape. The gym is a stone's throw from here and, he could train me for the "selection", he says.

"It's clean, cheap, but… is gym good for your health?" he asks me.

Yes, I believe it can be good for me.

Physical activity has always been good for me.

I am a former athlete, after all, "former" because, despite several sports I practiced during the following years of my competitions, I consider track and field as the most beautiful and important sport activity which I lovingly practiced between the Seventies and the Eighties. I was a sprinter and I have also been Italian champion of relay race 4 x 100, during those years. I am really proud of myself.

What a healthy living and how many happy memories teenage years leave with you!

In the 1970s, believe me, and whoever lived those years knows that, it was almost inconceivable that you didn't drink, smoked, nor even had a joint or played the guitar. Whereas for me it was like that.

Except for the guitar that I liked strumming near the fire, on the beach, in the evening, I was a pure girl.

As if this was the price I had to pay I didn't have a high consideration at school, among my classmates, my "friends".

I was the "weirdo", "the little Arabian girl", who rarely spoke and who, on coming out of school, walked to the "field" for training.

"It is better not to invite her to the parties... she is a nuisance!

She does not even smoke."

Then after lots of years I have been greatly re-evaluated while, most of them, had "lost" themselves in their own troubles and... didn't make it.

So finally I didn't make it as well and sent it one more text.

Silence.

Web search engine: Dragonfly.

Libellulus (*Librettuccio= Booklet*)

It is an insect belonging to the order Odonata, insects that are biologically linked to an aquatic environment, has got very big eyes, elongated abdomen, four spread and webbed wings just like a book .

Very fast in flight.

Only when adults they can "take flight" but spend their existence always around the water.

Splash splash.

Thoughts… in the outfield
"Thirty-year olders nowadays"

The famous thirty-years old crisis!
Well ... I wonder who can remember it.
But, on second thoughts ... I think:
"What a wonder generation, thirty-years old people today. Charming, full of good intentions but, eternally undecided, uncertain, fragile, and still unconscious.
So tender."

Thoughts… in the outfield
"The Journey"

How maddening!... Grrrr... when it mounts, you cannot control it.

As my mother used to say, I have a hot head and a cold heart.

I was a rebel for those times, although very introspective, quiet, reflective, I used to read, write and fluctuate into my inner world.

I loved art and when I had grown up, I would have liked to be a photo reporter, standing alone and independent… instead, here I am "government employee". I would have never wanted to depend on anyone, with a fixed-fool salary which doesn't make me meet ends, one month paid holiday per year, and, after all…I must consider myself lucky.

The only thing that can comfort me is that, however, I had a good time until I was thirty, since, at the age of eighteen I "ran away from home" to follow "the American Dream", to study and learn English, my passion for Eastern philosophy and Native Indians, free to travel, get to know, overstep the mark, discover new and different places, above all inside of me, trying to find, every time, everywhere, in every face, my own place in this world.

The journey is the real wealth.

You can easily recognize a person who has travelled extensively, or who loves traveling, as his eyes shine with a particular unclouded light ...

I am not talking about tourists package tours, they weren't really my thing.
I loved camping, nature, adventure, after all, I have always felt an "*Adventurewoman*".

9. "How to forget"

Finally I joined the gym, now I am "out of danger"…
but, "You must pay great attention to the axillary cavity
as it is very delicate", the technician on duty warns me.
She is very nice and immediately recognizes me,
although has seen me only once, at the beginning of my
treatment.
She welcomes me with a big smile and says: "Hello
beautiful, I was waiting right for you, hurry up, so today
we can go back home quite early. What a nice figure you
have… you are only two years younger than me but… I
look like your mother indeed"!
She has a strong Roman accent so she makes me laugh.
She reminds me my dear old friend Pedro, from Ostia
Lido.

Ostia is Rome's seaside, location of my teenage years, a
place that remained in my heart, and where we settled
after being "repatriated" from Africa, after the refugee
Camp, after the boarding-school… some memories get
there quite carved inside you.

How to forget the decorous tears shed by my sister and
I, when we were only nearly seven and nine years-old,
to the news, which we couldn't
yet understand, to have to live everything all of a sudden,
school, friends, home, the loved small room, our toys…
"No, not our toys"! "Each one of you can take only one
doll" said mom, with a sad and throaty voice.

How to forget

the face of my younger sister, at Customs, when a big and fat soldier approached her and, sarcastically whispered: "What a nice doll... can I stroke it?"

She was a naïve child so... she held tightly her dolly while screaming: "Don't come closer to my doll... my mom told me not to make anyone touch it!"

Ta-bum!

He ripped away from her hands her dear doll she used to talk with, comb and get dressed as if it was her daughter. Then he detached its head to check if we had hidden something inside. Some women were obliged to loose their "chignon", a very fashionable hairdo in the 1970s, but this is a funny memory.

Anyway I have been more crafty.

So... taking advantage of my agility and cunning, just holding tight to my chest my favourite dolly, I passed under the iron bar which divided the borders, after which ... there was freedom, and I, faster than the speed of light, was already on the other side.

I ran, ran and I could feel my heart beat quite crazy in the chest...

I am still very excited just thinking about it.

But finally, my loved dolly and I, succeeded in doing it.

I was so proud of me.

How to forget

The boat, the feeling of a "rip-off" and, printed inside my mind, the image of me, between the hands of my mother and my sister with tears streaming down our face, while looking at our homeland getting further and further in the horizon until it disappeared.

How to forget
the Refugee Camp, in Alatri, near the Castles of Rome.
There we felt like being in a concentration camp.
I came back there some time ago, after 37 years, and it still looks like that.
That experience left a great pity and sadness in my heart.
Four people living in a room of about 20 square meters, very cold, although it was late summer, inside huge stone barracks, with bathrooms situated outside, 50 meters away.
But these were, mostly, the problems of grown-ups.
For us children, all little cousins, that was a big "playground", where we could run, invariably skinned off our knees, climb, pick up the blackberries and every time we came back home with our hands and pockets full of "gems" of a particular rock that shines in the mountains of that Country.
Stones that my mother promptly cast away screaming:
"There is no room for us here, there is no need for stones at all!"
We spent a few months there, too many according to my mother.

And how can I forget
my first meeting with Rome… the boarding-school, the "Children's Home" or something like that, a kind of former Orphanage, that was not really "former".
There I attended the fourth year of Primary school.
From Monday to Friday I had lessons with the "Maidens" in the morning, but only after having made the beds and cleaned the toilets (I can't absolutely forget the lost expression of my younger sister, in front of

her undone bed, crying: "I am not able to make my bed" …and so, every morning, I hurried up for making mine and then hers too).

Then at twelve o'clock: lunch break.

All of us had to wear a blue uniform, with white shirt and socks, to go to the Refectory table and saying our prayers, that nuns forced us to perform everytime before sitting down.

Afternoon: homework time. Then, playtime.

An old little basketball pitch, or maybe so it had been once, where we loved playing ball and having goodtime. It was surrounded by a wire netting, to prevent us from running, as lots of orphans occasionally tried to do it.

In fact one day, a boy, asked me to run away with him just saying: "I don't give a damn… as I have no parents"! But fortunately I have my parents.

Anyway I was in his debt, because, despite himself, he taught me the value of family.

Every Saturday night was special as we were allowed to watch TV. At that time, I believe, there was the television programme "*Canzonissima*" and also the famous *Raffaella Carrà*… we were so happy. Except when the "Maidens" punished me for not having eaten or for having thrown the bread away to eat only the chocolate… so I was obliged, before watching TV, to clear all the tables (and they were a lot!). It seemed to be in one of those movies where there are long tables with lots of children, locked up in orphanage or, if they are lucky, in a convent, that was the same.

And, as it was not enough: "And no television tonight, after dinner you must go straight to bed!"

Gasp gasp, Sgrunt sgrunt.

And on "Holy Sunday": have a guess?
Of course to Church everybody.
Then, however, how fun!
After lunch, we were all in single line and down to walk
up until the artificial lake in Eur, a green area of Rome,
where, in its green fields, we enjoyed tumbling and
making somersaults.
How beautiful it was... a nice feeling of freedom, on our
body still unripe.
Sometimes, they took us to the Amusements Park…and
there It was wonderful.
Unforgettable memories.

And to put an end to these strange lines, as my friend
Pedro said, how can I forget his "poem" composed in
the late 1980's and dedicated to me? Well…

"To a Friend"

"Among all my friends,
one of them is so strange and so lovely
and binds me to my dear Gabry.
Well, strange because, among people,
Quite rarely befall
that a man and a woman are friendly,
It's like to serve anchovies with candy.
Since men only think about getting laid,
and they only love hitting on maid…
While women, well… they are something else,
Friendship to them,
Is to feel, and be felt in reverse.
In the game of life, it is well-known,

there is people who sweet-talk and say:
"Men and Women, they are the same"…
but after just having a glance or getting a whiff …
they reveal their hidden cards… only a bluff.
I sometimes think about this,
yes, about my friendship with Gabry.
She is very womanly, but some kind of brawny,
she surely can wear trousers and skirt as well,
or better, I would like to state that she is so smart,
and given the same conditions,
she has more nuts than men in any case.
Obviously men have got them, they feel the whole,
but if you just could strip their briefs,
and open the nuts up indeed,
you would not find anything!"
And to put an end to these strange lines
written down quite roughly here in the kitchen,
I would like to close with a rhyme …
Being friend of a woman does not require all that,
but at the same time you have to get
that, before being a woman,
she is, above all, a human!" [2]

Pedro

---

[2] Original text: "Tra tutte l'amicizie che ciò io,/c'è una n'sacco strana,
n'sacco bella,/è quella che me lega a Gabriella./Ho detto strana perché, tra
la gente,/non è cosa poi c'accade normalmente,/che n'omo cò 'na donna
siano amici,/è come servì er dolce cò l'alici./Perché noantri semo limitati a
c…. f…../e annassene pè prati…/mentre 'e donne , mbè tutt'artra cosa,/pè
loro l'amicizia solitamente,/vo dì sentisse si, ma veramente./Ner gioco
della vita è risaputo,/c'è gente con le dita di velluto che dice: "L'omo e la
donna? Semo pari…/ ma basta n'colpo d'occhio e n'po' de fiuto… /pè faie
scoprì 'e carte, tutti bari./Gni tanto io ci penso a sta storiella,/sì, insomma,

10. "BIRI"
A paw to heart

Gulp! Two years!?!
Two years went by!
The faithful, unique, real companion of my life: Birillo, Biri
for friends. Unique in his kind as all loved dogs.
My old and tired Biri left me on a nasty and painful
Saturday, after fifteen years of "fusion", my natural end,
with a proud look full of love until the last sigh.
We grew up together.
He taught me more than how I did with him.
We often should take animals as example.
Dogs not only are a good company, but you can interact,
talk, cry and laugh with them. We learn to care and respect,
and… yes, we pick up lots of shit I know, but, above all, tons of love.
My Biri has seen lots of things in fifteen years of life.
He was always with me, ready to follow me everywhere,
to wipe my tears, to console my delusions, to lick my
wounds, and to give me always his paw, or better, his

---

a st'amicizia, a Gabriella./E' na ragazza n'gamba, n'sacco donna,/che porta
bene pantaloni e gonna./Vorrebbi dì, pè famme capì mejo,/che è n'gamba
e, spesso, a pari condizioni,/ rispetto a n'omo, lei c'ha più cojoni./ In senso
metaforico, si intende, l'omo ce l'ha davero, se li sente ma, se dovessi
tojeie 'e mutanne e/ aprije li cojoni veramente… a tanti dentro n'troveresti
gnente!/E pè dì fine a sti versetti strani,/ scritti n'fretta qua n'cucina,/ vojo
conclude cò na frase a rima…/P'esse amico a 'na donna ce vo poco ma, ar
tempo stesso tanto, si n'te sona che, prima/ d'esse donna è na persona!"//

hand on my heart.

"It seems trivial, but now,
he is probably enjoying
This beautiful sky",
A friend of mine wrote down that day.
"Light is boundless,
drops of silver fall down from the sky ...
Up there, probably they are celebrating
something important, the arrival of a newcomer
a very special guest."
"So there's more love than ever today, up there,"
I replied.
Over the life
beyond the matter
and death itself.
Thanks Biri.

It is impossible not to note down the telegrams and letters that the children who loved Biri very much, sent me as they were really sorrowful since he passed away ...
Right to smile a bit... I'll write out their messages quite literally:

"Dear Birillo,
When you died, your owner Gabbriella was very sorrowful.
When the sad news of your death was anounced to us we were very unhappy and so we wrote out firstly a telegram and then a letter for you and another one for your magnificent owner.
Telegram:

All of us cry: "Be strong Gabbriella, as the small and tender Biri will be forever in both your and our heart".

Love for Biri, by Laura, Maria Palma, Daniela, Stefano, Tania, Peter, Sabbrina and Lucia.

Letter for Biri:

Dear Biri,
Since you're not longer in this world,
things have changed. Your owner is not as happy as she used to be.
The day you passed away, she was very desolate and we must say we also suffered greatly. Biri you were a beautiful and brilliant dog.
Your owner loves you very much so she always brings you flowers.
Now, my dear Biri, I have to leave you.
Goodbye by Daniela and all the others.

Letter for Gabbriella:

"Dear Gabbriella,
I had a dog as well, but he died too because in this world there are lots of bad people who don't realize what you feel when an animal dies.
You have suffered so much and me too, but when my dog died I took another one and so I forgot everything. I hope you too will act in the same way."

The wisdom of children!

11. "One step away"

I'm excited, like a teen-ager.
After waiting in vain, unanswered questions, dashed hopes, finally I can embrace its wings.
If I were an emotion... I would be a palpitation.
And the dense rain, falling today, is tears of joy.
How to describe an emotion?
Well, shaking hands, heart beating, quite crazy indeed with thousand beats per minute, so that you are frightened that it could also be visible from your shirt, and then you feel like a moron, all your securities, your poise and self-control get lost, disappear when they face a real emotion.
But, how can we fight or cancel it as well?
It's like having an itchy part of your body but you cannot scratch, or like trying to look but being unable to see, or like touching something that you cannot feel.
So my brain reminds me of when I fell in love for the first time and I coined a strange term as it was defined, "the *Blassenses*", the blast of all five senses:

The *Blassight*, the blast of sight
The *Blastouch*, the blast of touch
The *Blasearing*, the blast of hearing
The *Blasmell*, the blast of smell
The *Blastaste*, the blast of taste.

I used to say that I would have got married only with the man who would be able to make me feel all the five

senses in the same time in a perfect harmony... in every sense, with all my own senses.
In fact, I am still single.
Youth delirium.

Now that I think about it, I am pretty sure that the friendly Ciccillo told me: "After the tenth you must get a blood test done to control the azotemia and glycaemia. We must regularly check the concentration of white blood cells", the new doctor adds while giving me the prescription "You know, the radiation is dangerous for red blood cells" .
It's just a colour matter, I think.

I turn on the stereo and smile…
"One step away
from all I want
and I know it's all here" .

"There is no more appropriate song", I think.

Music often plays these tricks.

12. "Free Will"

So brief, just a few words, essential "my Dragonfly".
Probably I have upset its "regularity", made both its certainties and values falter, the same values in which I greatly believe myself, so… I can't blame it for this.
I read somewhere that "absolute love does not foresee neither falls, nor defeats… it only grants the soul and makes fun of cowards who don't dare deeds which are great"…
And brave as well, I might add.
Maybe it takes both courage and strength to follow your heart, always. Moreover, the saying is: "Follow your heart", not your rationality.
To choose what is right for you, despite who says "This is wrong", to prefer the "normal" because the other one is "unusual", or the white as the other one is black, the peace and security of your "nest", rather than the etherealness and the risk of a new emotion.
Free will.
It is like playing a game, you can either win or lose, there is always a risk, but you are the only one to decide whether to face and go on playing or give everything up.
The famous "middle way" cannot exist in a real game, either you fly or you crash to the ground.
You can take a step back and look at the vortex that spins around and you can't neither stop it, nor separate it, or you can get off the carousel at the next round, since you know that there will be others with new faces,
new stories, new emotions… it's the game of life.
Eyes, though, don't lie.

So my selfish longing for love clings right to that glance, until the deepest of my heart, where there are no limits, rules or borders at all.

Ciccillo is thoughtful and very paternal today,
unlikely his colleague, a woman who is a bit more detached and professional. It's the two of them who take care of me so I feel very important.
She, however, does not appear to be in a good mood, as she reproaches Ciccillo continuously, she is strict, accurate and, after calibrating everything to the last detail, and giving me the usual warnings... do you know that soft tickle, when you have bronchitis, which affects you when lying down?
Well, I felt that and the fear of a cough crept inside me, I tried every way to control the breath while saying to myself: "Don't cough, don't cough, don't cough…"
Then I coughed.
Stragulp!
You can imagine her gaze.
So she came back and balanced me once again after pressing, with excessive force for my liking, a kind of black marker there, in the middle of my chest, "To reinvigorate the color of the tattoo" says, then she adds "When you wash yourself it fades, unfortunately the underneath one never goes away!"
Why did she need to remind me of that?
Then she returns to her "nest" puffing, while I feel the echo of her words: "Come on, Ciccì this is the last one, so we can go back home quite soon tonight."
Mumble mumble...
She reminds me of someone ...

13. "The dancing little nerve"

Let's say I have been living all sorts in my life, as they say, and I am aware of being a courageous and fearless woman, but to see or rather to get my skin "penetrated" with a needle, is something that I have always been puzzled about.

I hate the idea of something sharp that perforates the skin and the underlying layers. I never loved the "fashion" of piercing, I get puzzled by all those holes in ears now worn out, noses, even on tongue and nipples, and I don't want to add where else… it is better not to say.

Anyway I like tattoos, not obviously those that I had done here, but I mean the artistic drawings rich in intimate meanings, some of them looking like real works of art.

On my skin I have two of them symbolizing my stars: Libra and Buffalo, although lots of people are pretty sure that an "even number" brings bad luck. I was thinking to have a third tattoo done, quite small like the others, and delicate. But now, if we actually count the three "tatoos" they made me here, I have five of them, so… it's an add number and let's not mention it anymore.

Our protagonist today is: "the dancing little nerve".

Oh, what a coincidence, as soon as I lie down, *traktrum*, something occurs to me. Nothing strange happens for twenty-three hours and 55 minutes, but why does it happen exactly during those five minutes?

Well, imagine you suddenly have eyelid beats that can't just stop… it was the same but on the legs. So firstly began my left leg to shake and the technician from his "box" told me by microphone: "Gabriella, don't move please!"

Eh, I would like it too. Then my right leg, quite jealous of the other one, began to tremble as well … so that it seemed to be the Symphony Orchestra show.

He was desperate and did not know what to tell me.

I anyway was more desperate than him, while attempting in vain to keep them steady. The "treatment" lasted more than usual today ... thank goodness I am off for the weekend.

"To you who are, just you are
substance of my days,
substance of my dreams"...

I love this song and *"Tell it to the Marines"*.

Thoughts… in the outfield
"Magnetic Attraction"

"The hedgehog that clams up…
and the Dragonfly that flies away".
Sent.
"Flying but not hedgehog".
It replies.
Gulp… mumble mumble...

It is a magnetic attraction
that creates a motion in my mind,
your skin,
your shyness
your energy,
your moist eyes, in whose tears
I would like to dive.
I can feel you in the air I breath,
as a smell that surrounds me,
inebriates and possesses me.
I can feel you like a swirling wave
breaking into the rocks,
or like a drum rolling relentlessly.
I feel you in the wind …
softly caressing the silence.
I can feel you,
desert, so far away mirage.

Thoughts… in the outfield
"Memories… dusting off my inner memory drawers"

Once someone wrote me: "I have two memories of you:
A) an adorable, sweet, sensitive, friendly, sincere person who loves to give a lot of herself;
B) a proud iceberg."
Yes, this is me.
"Beautiful things never last too long", I said…
"No, beautiful things can last forever in the memory of who lived them."
And I learned the lesson.
One day I found a ticket on the windscreen of my car:
"I see that you are at home and I am looking at your window with great melancholy. I would like to look into your eyes for whispering what I never dared say to you. But if you like, I will patiently wait for you every night. In the meantime, I can live on a memory."
P.s.
"If you want to know who I am, you can listen to the voice of your consciousness (but you haven't got it)."

Wow... I wonder how I may have hurt this human being. But who was it, by the way? I never knew it. Maybe it is a consequence of the eternal law of cause and effect, "what goes around, comes around" or better, "life is a circle", I also had my fair amount of pain, sufferings and betrayals too, and the following letter can be an example of that:

"Dear Gabry

if you consider a fault to have some problems or not being able to find an inner balance, then forgive me, but my only fault, maybe, is to have a great confusion inside myself … In the past two years with you, full of moments more or less happy anyway, you have filled a few gaps inside me, you have watered my roots allowing me to be more stable in the ground, your words will be always for me stimulus for reflection, your face a reason for sweetness.

You are the woman I loved you most, although I showed it to you least of all.

For all evil you have to go through Gabry, never change thanks to my stupid being, but go your way and don't look back.

You are miles ahead of me, believe me.

You are the one who says: "True love is the medicine against all evil", well, you are lucky as you know how to love and this will help you during your wonderful life's journey.

Gabry, don't throw yourself away, don't throw away what so many people, me included, would give their own soul for".

I love you, M.

14. "Technology"

In the Blue Room, the TV is on, with the volume up and to be honest, I feel a little bit annoyed.

Maybe it is because of the general election.

During the elections everything changes... but later everything comes back to normal.

And sometimes things get even worse.

In addition to the usual ones, today there are new faces, so this is a new adventure for them. Beside me a man fell asleep while waiting... I wonder how he can sleep with this chaos.

I have not met a young face yet since I started my treatment and, I must say that, despite my green age, I feel so young here.

And these women make me feel a sense of protectiveness, since they remind me of my mother.

I feel so peaceful today, despite its silence.

Cellular phones are like this, they always make you wait for something, a text message, every kind of sign or thought, and if they do not arrive you feel so deluded.

I know, as I experienced it on my skin, that you do not have to expect anything from anybody.

"Everything that comes is something more", I say.

But anyway you are always disappointed about it.

Everything was quite different before, we did not have these troubles, mobile phones did not exist and when you went out, it was really impossible to reach you.

You expected nothing, since nothing could arrive, but

you were more peaceful indeed.

The greatest problem could be "The quest for the lost coin"anyway if you had it, you had to be lucky, first to find a phone booth and, then to find a phone inside it (sometimes there was a phone inside the box but it was faulty or… "false alarm… without the receiver!").

However, I don't know how, but we could meet as well and we were so happy and lighthearted.

At that time computers did not exist so, we used to write long letters… how beautiful it was… it is not possible to explain the emotion of receiving a letter from a friend or a lover too.

It tasted different.

Well, letters have to fight against both time and distance but these obstacles can give them a different flavour.

The pleasure of waiting.

You know that your words are already travelling through loose sheets which drive a soul towards another.

A pleasure that, by now, we have lost with email and short messages.

Fortunately there is my flatmate who helps me to solve every IT problem. She is so "technological" and has a remarkable skill with I-pod, Mp3 players, Software, Hardware, I-Phone, I-Tunes, Bluetooth and so on.

I am just a self-taught, like in every situations of my life. I tried to steal lots of its secrets and I partly succeeded in doing this, but I am like a "lone surfer" who just takes only what he feels can enrich his boundless thirst for knowledge and his unsatisfied hunger for emotions, in an endless quest in the search engine of life.

15. "Let there be Chaos... Not Quiet"

Rare, microscopic fragments of your time granted to me.
But how can we quench our thirst with so few drops of water?
Thank goodness my daily appointment and the bicycle ride free me of such questions.
Even the sky is gloomy, like my thoughts.

Therapy, instead, went smoothly, and ran like clock-work, the new technician was quite silent and brisk.
His only words were: "Don't move by any means now"... and "you can put your arms down". Good evening and thank you. Anyway I didn't feel very talkative, today.
Fortunately my blood test results are good, figures are average, I am a small rock!
Today I am exactly half way of my progress and my skin holds out the treatments very well; "you're lucky to have dark skin, since is more resistant and less del cate"... after all, in many respects, it is always "just a skin matter."

My flatmate came back... you notice it from the "notquiet" mess in our flat.
The violin is somewhere, the scores are somewhere else, handbags, suitcases, iron, lots of clothes in the washing-machine, other clothes hanged out to dry, etc... but now, I am accustomed to this chaos.
She is an artist, sensitive and very distracted indeed, and I am very fond of her for this reason too. She came back

home more serene than how she was before leaving, because of her "love afflictions". But she is a thirty-year older of nowadays too, with her confusion, her doubts, spasmodically searching for her inner balance.

We talked very much, like we had not done for a while, since she was completely involved in her own love story. "Now you're in a limbo" I say to her, a bit like me too.

After all, love stories resemble each other, with their implacable mechanisms that keep repeating over time.

Sometimes love is an awful feeling, it makes you blunder, or makes you feel bad indeed.

But sometimes it makes you conciliate with the all world.

16. "Emotions"

Adri left once again and in the house there are both tidiness and quiet now.

Well, to be honest, tidiness is a little bit exaggerated, I would say it is jumble that actually belongs to me, just like on my mind.

I know I'm a sufficiently balanced and quite strong woman, especially when I have to face the most difficult heavy and painful problems of life.

The harder they are, the stronger I react.

Life is tough, but I am tougher.

I love myself.

After years of introspectiveness and studies on myself, I realized that my biggest problem, or rather the stumbling rock where I always crash myself is of emotions one.

I am unable to manage my emotions.

It drives me crazy.

I am not always able to protect myself and not allow the loved person to enter myself and scratch my soul.

My dancing little nerve came back once again, just today when there is the same strict and pedantic doctor of the other day on duty.

I can't believe it.

Today, however, he is in a good mood and also addresses me a wisecrack, like: "Hey beautiful, if you get fatter, in a bit you will be unable to lie on this couch"... Ha ha ha!

He is a bundle of fun!

I am having dinner at my parents'.

Mom is an excellent cook and has prepared something good for me, this woman always grabs me by the throat. What would I do without her!

17. "The Sound of Silence"

The first one was on March 17th.
The journey where the lips are the world map.
And then the infinite embrace that tunes the breaths.
AMonththatlookslikeaDaythatlookslikeaYear.
I would always have liked very much to write a song, set
it to music and play it as well by my Sax (which by now
will be full of cobwebs), under the window of my
beloved, right like a serenade...
I am a past-time woman.
I have been always quite pleased to meet a real "gentle-
man" who can say: "After you, please" or who opens the
door for you, gives you flowers, takes you out and pays
for dinner too. Sometimes I like to direct the game, I am
intrigued by the idea of being able to turn a situation
upside down, just creating particular atmospheres and
upset all the glazed that were quietly set on me first.
I like people who firmly knows how to direct a game,
feeling the exhilaration of being a woman among emotions, glances and wise arms. Like in every comparison,
where the reversals are essential to keep the balance of
opposing forces.

Sometimes silence may become so heavy, so heavy as to
compress your heart.

"My thought flies to you...
to reach the images
carved already into consciousness

like everlasting emotions
that I can't forget anymore…
Every time I will feel you distant
Every time I would like to talk to you
Right for saying that you are the only
most important thing for me"…

Another musical poem appropriate to the moment.

Also my head is heavy today, in the Blue Room.
Maybe it is the weather, the sky is white with some scattered puffs and it is drizzling…
Maybe it depends on these neon lights turned on expressly for this gloomy day or, perhaps, always because of the silence…
I don't know… mumble mumble...
It's my turn and be it so.

18. "Forbidden Fruit"

I often wonder why mankind and, particularly, women always love running after the "forbidden fruit".
The more it is difficult to reach it, unlikely, mysterious, impossible, the more we like it.
I've never understood the reason.
Perhaps, after all, all of us are a little bit masochistic.
A man who is kind, polite, helpful, we don't like, and we think he is quite a bore. I have always heard that "In love, winner is the one who flees", but what a cruel law! Why must we flee?
Wouldn't it be better to discuss, clarify and then... "the proof of the pudding is in the eating", otherwise... no hard feelings.
But sometimes it is quite difficult indeed.
We must bring into it all the complications, inner problems, guilt, fears, desires, torments.
Nevertheless... the woman is the greatest mystery in the universe. From the top of the awareness that I have reached, I generally face it up, as for better or for worse, if I like you, I say it right to you or somehow I show it, anyway if I don't like you I show and say my dislike as well, even harder.
I learned to be more honest with myself and with others too and this makes me feel better.
I hate those who run away without a word, without having at least the courage to face you and tell what they think about you on your face. Cowards!
Not to mention friends... They always leave you right

whenever you most need them.

It almost seems, a law of nature.

But I'm not like that, I am different.

Or at least, I have never been like that till now.

Maybe it depends on the good breeding I received, (my parents are so friendly and welcoming that they would sleep on the floor just to make their guests feel more comfortable), maybe it's in our genes, I don't know, but I am really unable to deny my help to a friend who is in difficulty.

Since I was a young girl, my mother reprimanded me: "Here she is the missionary, always friendly and ready for people's needs... then, when you need them... they all disappear. Don't be foolish like your mother, get wise, bite or you will be eaten up"...

She was so right!

I've tried it hard, and I sometimes still try it, but this is my nature and there is nothing I can do about it.

Two frightened faces, in the Blue Room, maybe this is the first time for them, it is undoubtedly clear.

I stop writing to observe them.

One of them is sitting motionless, rigidly, obese even if quite young, with a black scarf on her head (and the reason is obvious) she has a sad, scared and also disheartened face. I would almost like to console her... (here is my missionary spirit that occasionally resurfaces), but she doesn't give me any signal.

The other one, instead, is standing, quite upset, and seems like begging for my help with her eyes.

I smile at her and, as if she was waiting just for this, she comes closer and I feel her strong need of talking, of giving vent to her own emotions.

So I let her do it.

I listen to her for a long time, "I am fifty-eight years old and I am so lonely" she starts telling me.

"This adventure made me closer to faith, to God, it is my only foot hold" ... Then they call her, it is her turn, but in her face, now more relaxed, it seems rising a smile.

Thoughts… in the outfield
"AdventureWomen"

I have always been fascinated by airports.

That coming and going of people, crossing of destinies everybody with their suitcases full of hopes, dreams, illusions, "desires to move", to discover different and remote places.

A journey, sometimes towards a known place, but often towards the unknown.

I greeted Maja and Titti this morning, from the big family of "AdventureWoman", destination Kuala Lumpur.

They have been chosen, among many of us, coming from all over Italy, to realize a week report "in the footsteps" of the official expedition that came back from Malaysia just a month ago. It was a great emotion to see them laugh full of pride and enthusiasm.

This year we are going to celebrate the twentieth anniversary of "Adventure Woman" foundation:a Voyage, a "distinct world", an extraordinary experience conceived and carried out by an "Adventure genius" that, every year, gives to a carefully chosen team made up by six courageous and lucky women, the opportunity to cover, for a hundred days, thousands of kilometers in remote and fascinating places, right driving famous off-road vehicles, like "pick up", or with any other necessary means as well: horse, bicycle, canoe, Tibetan bridge, etc…

Women, who must be able to fight with spirit of sacrifice and determination, to overcome with strength and intelligence all arduous obstacles involved in those kind of travels; "hard work" which will be then repaid by the beauty of landscapes, the majesty of nature, by the attractive taste for adventure, the infinite sensations felt and the fantastic images later reported.

We met, or rather "recognized", thanks to this "magic world" and together with the mythical "Roman women group", we immediately loved one other!

Good luck girls...

Special Women, or rather "AdventureWomen".

Thoughts... in the outfield
"The Language of the Universe"

The common tendency, typically, is to point the finger at others for anything or for every mistake committed.

It is easier and it helps you to lighten your own conscience.

Anyway the others are only the mirror of ourselves.

But it is quite difficult to question our own assumptions. The pain that comes from the outside, from others, ought to be a stimulus for speculation, a lesson as well. Maybe you can discover some of our faults among the lines of this pain or, it is possible to understand something negative to avoid.

The cycles of nature are simple and immense, we only have to decode the language of the universe ... I burn, I withdraw myself. Danger, estrangement.

Easy, isn't it?

19. "The Anniversary"

Remark:
"When your great-niece, daughter of your younger sister's daughter, comes to life...
When your parents celebrate forty-eight years of marriage...
When guys begin to call you "Madam"...
Does it mean that you are getting older?
And today, it is the anniversary of my "old ones".
I gave them a little present with a greeting card :

"To my Parents,
my origins,
my roots,
my blood,
my heart,
my greatest Love".

I know that my mother was very touched.
My father... well, maybe he was moved as well, but he doesn't show it.
We went to Fiumicino, a little seaside city, to eat some good fish.
My mom was so happy, the two of us also got drunk, with wine and lemoncello; but for my father, more rational, it looked like was an ordinary day indeed.
Apparently nothing can move him, neither birth, nor death, not even special occasions, or maybe... except only for "dancing". My parents met dancing and they

have been going on doing it for fifty years as well.
It's the only thing that he loves apart from football.
And all the rest seems quite unnecessary.
I love him because he is my father.
But, whenever I see them dancing together, with their tender grey hair, they really touch my heart.

And here, in the Blue Room the images are confused today, perhaps the lemoncello is a party to this, who knows...
I look out the window, the sun is shining, but it is unable to warm my heart up.
Silence reigns above everything.
And the effects, slowly begin to be felt... I can deeply feel it all over my skin.

20. "I always want to say Yes!"

I like the radio.
I often listen to it, when I am at home, in my car, it is an
excellent company and I couldn't do without it.
Music can always help you, it is your advisor and gives
you support, courage and also makes you cry.
Music can do everything.
And before leaving I listen to the last notes:

"I will change the life that, can't change me…
I will change the life that,
that disillusioned me more than you"…
There are songs, such as people that more
than others remain attached to your soul,
imprinted on your skin.
Not by chance… I find a small piece of paper,
Looking inside my backpack:
"I always want to say yes…
to the aperitifs with friends,
to unexpected invitations
to evenings until late,
to sweaty sessions at the gym,
to art exhibitions,
to dinner with friends,
to tours by motorbike,
to the evenings at the cinema,
to theatrical performances,
to every kind of music,
to my dream trips,

to all my passions
I always want to say yes"!

And I also reply yes to the echo of my name, not exactly whispered by the technician on duty.
"You are the last one, as usual, but meanwhile you go on writing and do not realize the time passing"… then giggle and next one, please. "He is right", I think.
Writing distracts me to such an extent that I remain almost Bothered in having to stop writing, when it is my turn.
The room is full, today.
The blue chairs have been already taken, all of them are full of lives just upset.
I feel observed myself, for the first time.
I have already put almost forty signatures, bureaucracy also hangs over here quite dutifully, like the rain that today flows very unrelentingly, sweet companion of my thoughts.
"Reddened skin, you ought to use more lotion", recommends the Doctor, "Anyway, it is less than many other women, so you're very lucky to have dark skin".
Ok.

21. "Thank God there is the Sun!"

The silence was broken, shattered, and my dream crashed, got scattered. Maybe the silence was better, as it leave you with hope at least, an illusion, even if... I am a practical person and I prefer a word to a coward silence.

I also know that, when we fall down, we can rise up stronger than ever as well, and we get more careful than before.
My mother, like every mother does with her children, always told me, trying to comfort me:
"When one door closes, a big gate opens".
Many doors have been shut in the meantime, but as for the gate... not even a shadow!
Maybe, we sometimes create our own world, false myths or imaginary movies with incredible and passionate stories, outcome of our deepest desires, but then, when we put our feet back on the ground, we must accept the harsh reality, the changeable nature of feelings, the mere evidence.
If we only could control our crazy heartbeat, our wandering mind that floats everywhere but, at the end, always comes back there again.
It is so, if you think so.
"Unfold your wings and fly up...
where I cannot reach you...
"You flow like the water,
and like the water you slide away

without almost any trace,
illusions of craziness with no outcome,
to then find ourselves alone …
Like the water you slide,
like the water you flow away"…

The room is half-empty.
"It is quite strange", I think, "the same feeling as my body", that feeling of emptiness that you feel whenever life rips you off of something very important and precious for you, whenever you feel alone and abandoned. Also the doctor noticed this, "Is there something wrong?", he asks me, "You're so quiet".
"Maybe it is hormones' fault" I reply, without any desire to smile.
Thank God there is the sun!
A breath of oxygen and tomorrow is a new day, who will live, will see.
After all, how my sweetest Adventure friend Babbi wisely says: "It doesn't take much… it's easy!"

22. "Life is a Puzzle"

By now, I tune up in unison with this Blue Room.
Today it is completely empty.
I look around and I feel unique.

Despite everything, I believe that in addition to basic needs, a healthy physical activity and a little bit of "Sense of humor" are the cure for all ailments.
I see lots of people get depressed, quite down, who lock themselves at home and withdraw.
But what is the use of it?
Why do they add sufferings to sufferings, why don't they look for the bright side of everything (because it is there).
"The devil is not always at one door", I believe it is right.
Difficult experiences must strengthen, not weaken you, we must never give up to the "Force test" of life, we must always fight and try to overcome them.
I often use to say:
"I stagger but don't give up".
Every experience, as beautiful or ugly that it can be, adds an important bit to your life.
It's like in a puzzle, where every piece, that you add, allows to understand the final artwork better.
But above all, we must protect, take care and pamper ourselves and, why not, love ourselves as well.

"Bless you that succeed in doing this", tells me quite

disheartened the "sadeyeswoman"... "I can't make it, nothing stimulate me to go on, I'm always at home, I don't even have a family, or a shoulder to cry on".

So I give her mine, even if it is very tiny, while she, grateful, smiles and offers me a cup of coffee.

She waited for me outside right for this reason, how tender!

I felt her deepest gratitude on my skin, and it made me feel better. She also did something for me, after all.

It is always just a skin matter.

In a world made up of "greatness", full of expectations, sometimes, it takes very little, a piece at the right place and the game is played. That's it!

Thoughts… in the outfield
"Utopia"

When I was already a far-seeing teenager, I used to write about friendships:
"It's one of the sweetest caresses for the heart, one of the most delicate happiness for the soul, anyway, it has got only a weak point… it's so rare!"
"Relief and support in this life is to have a person whom you can open your heart to, tell each other intimate things to entrust and the inner secrets of your soul, which you keep jealously secreted to the eyes of indifferent people, or to have a person who, in the happy circumstances rejoices by your side and in difficulty can give you support."
A utopia!

Thoughts... in the outfield
"As a Work of Art"

A suggestion...
Taking the cue from the great Chaplin:

"Live as you believe,
do what your heart tells you,
what you feel like doing.
 "Life is a play that does not allow testing.
So, sing, cry, dance, laugh and live intensely,
before the curtain is closed and the piece ends
with no applause."

Thoughts come and go... life is like this.

23. "Female Energy"

When I was a child I used to love writing my diary.
And I went on doing this until I was about twenty-five years old.
It was my dearest friend, intimacy companion, my "imaginary friend".
I used to bring it with me all the time, everywhere, and write curled into my little world. I was a very shy, introverted and silent girl, I used to love listen to music, read and write, especially my diary, but also poems and songs as well. That was my own way to express myself, my need to take out, somehow, what, inside my soul, there was (above all at that age!), otherwise I felt like going off.
It made me grow up, just giving me more self-confidence, self-esteem and awareness, just opening the doors of the "other's" world for me.
I must have kept my diaries, in some remote corner of the basement, I guess...
They have been there for more than twenty years, locked into a leather suitcase, perfect "migrant" style and...I think it is time to take them out and dust them off.
It will be both strange and funny to read about my past, my first teenage emotions, it will be a stimulus to make, somehow, sleepy memories resurface, the written proof of changes and mutations that time and experience caused in myself.
It is a little revival of my life.
Cool!
Better than introspection!

Better than psychoanalysis!

Working and really tiring weekend.
The only positive note was the arrival of my sister from Sicily with her daughters and granddaughter. How big my grandniece became!
She is only seven months old and she is trying to stand on her feet already.
It is a great emotion to see my niece breast-feed her.
Not to mention my sister, who looks like a woman in her thirties, and the thought she is already a grandmother seems to me so weird.
Time passes by inexorably.
The family is gathered, we are six daughters and only one man, daddy, that obviously succumbs to such a great female energy.
His regret is that he never had nor a male son or grandson at all, even if, the first child whom unfortunately my mother aborted, was a boy.
Then I was born.
Born and grown up among women, with women, thanks to women.
I never met my granddads but I had a wonderful and protective grandmother who, unfortunately, left us prematurely, the day of my tenth birthday… Sigh, sigh...
The other grandmother, instead, from my father's side, is over ninety years old and she lives in Sicily. It is very different, by the way I love her. Whenever she sees me, she says that I am her favourite granddaughter, (she has about a hundred grandchildren and great-grandchildren) but, I am pretty sure, that she says the same to all of us. And here's the "really nice" one today who greets me

with a big smile, "Hi beautiful, it's been a while since we last met, you look fine, come on… let's go and have a sun-bed"!

I smile at her and go towards my destiny, already so familiar to me.

24. "Love Hunger"

Sometimes words are not enough to express a state of mind, and this is one of those moments. I am not in the mood, but I will try to do it anyway.

It is raining outside.

It is by now an empathy with the weather.

I'm here with mom, she wanted to come with me after our mega-lunch with all the family.

Not even her worshipped granddaughters can distract her by her concern about me, I almost feel guilty.

"It's been a while since I last came with you... so I would like to come just for keeping you company".

So I decided to please her. I drive with a hand on the wheel, and the other one on her soft neck, thus caressing her.

I smile, increasingly grateful and hungry for her love.

Maybe it is my feeling, but her gaze change as she enters the Blue Room, a sad and melancholic veil draws down on her face.

It is something beyond description.

I cannot define through written words the boundless love I feel for her, every time, every day, more and more. It is an endless increasing.

Mother courage.

A real force of nature, my *Superadventuremom*.

The pedantic woman technician is on duty today and I really hope that nothing abnormal happens to me.

Today she is more talkative indeed, but anyway very professional, "Tomorrow is the last of those "normal" ones then you will have to talk with your doctor, who will explain you some trivialities"... "You will receive the last five treatments, those "special" ones with electrons, in Room A, next to this room".

"I hope I'll never see you again" .

"Only a suggestion, you ought to increase the dose of lotion, as your skin will burn a lot".

She, always so politely ruthless.

25. "The Bear Inside Me

Body muscles do have memory.

I experienced this on my skin.

After a long time of inactivity and, only three weeks of exercise, I must admit t I feel and look better, more toned, more vigorous, less lazy.

As I reckon I have become a little bit lazy over the years.

Despite I like being a "busy" woman, walking, cycling, playing sports, going to the seaside and above all travelling, my basic laziness, quite often, leads me to stay at home, and wallow in my own things.

I love spending evenings on my sofa, especially in winter, watching movies I like, downloading music and videos and, sometimes, even the *sweet idleness*.

To cut it short, I am like the bear that shuts itself up in its hut to enjoy honey, I just keep myself company and take good care of myself.

"Better alone than in bad company ", or rather, "If you want something done, do it yourself", my mother would say, since she is the Queen of sayings.

She has more than one trick up her sleeve.

And the first cycle of treatment has come to an end.

"You will start again within a week to do the last five, those special ones, as your skin needs a rest" Ciccillo says with a dejected and worried gaze because of my last "treatment" in his unit.

"Damn, you are so funny and you cheer me up, it's unusual to see people smiling here... I will miss you"...

"Well, I will come and see you sometimes" I reply with an immense tenderness in my heart.

And on the radio, on the way back, I get beats from: "A feeling matter", a real gem. I smile … music has always been my "partner in crime".

Around midnight...

It is my Biri's birthday, he would have turned seventeen today.

It is a while since this number has been persecuting me, well, it contains number seven, therefore everything is just fine.

That is part of my karma.

Happy birthday my little "blackblue" charming Prince!

["Flaming Break"]
Thoughts… in the outfield
"My Diaries"

And finally I dusted my diaries off, quite literally.
They were so full of dust to make me cough, but so full
of energy to move me so much.
The suitcase of memories.
Much of my past here quite handy, pages now yellowed
by time, yet so full of life.
From the diaries of a teenager:

"A friend made of paper is not enough"

"Dear diary, today I didn't have my usual training as it
was raining, so at about six p.m. I went to a party, but I
didn't have fun, and I don't even know the reason.
But why am I becoming like this?
I look like a parasite, I don't want to go out, I have no
fun, if only I find an explanation to all this, I could find
a solution too.
But how can I have all these problems being only sixteen...
and when I am fifty, what will I do?"
:)

That was the age of "never again" and "forever".

"Today one of my sister's girlfriends wrote a letter to my
boyfriend telling him she had fallen in love with him...

but how the heck can she loves if she is only thirteen-
years old and such a young girl... I don't have a clue!"
"He and I share a secret within the correspondence
between us...under the stamp we write sweet words,
secrets and intimate things that only we can read" ...

Mumble, mumble but... I wonder how large those
stamps were!!

"Poem"

"Me, you, the whole world
Let's stop for a moment only.
We breathe the same air
and walk on the same ground.
We eat in the same way
It's a same blood flowing inside of us.
We smell the same flowers
and look at the same sky.
We were conceived and were given birth as well.
We will conceive and give birth in identical way.
All of us need a night rest and, when we close
our eyes forever, we shall have an eternal sleep,
that will be identical as well!"

I don't think at that age I had already read "A spirit
level"
(A' livella) by Totò, the famous Italian actor, therefore,
I was just ahead.

"Dearest diary,
It is now the last day that I write to you, then I will pass

to your colleague both all my adventures and misadventures.

I'm sorry to leave you as I got very fond of you but, unfortunately, everything must come to an end one day or another and you, my dear friend, have come to an end as well".

:)

26. "Without any distinctions"

And here I am once again.

This time in the Room A, the one for "special treatments".

This is also blue.

After all, blue is a relaxing colour according to chromotherapy, and I always have loved it anyway. My mother tells me that, since I was a child, I have liked blue dresses very much and I also wanted my bedroom walls to be painted light blue with fluffy white clouds... maybe it was just a need of sea and sky.

I look around me. New faces, different, men and women of every class, shape, colour, but finally, here, we are all the same indeed, "certain things" don't spare anybody and don't make any distinctions, unlikely what people do. It's fair this way, even if the word fairness is really hard to comprehend and accept here.

The others shudder, are worried about schedules, "It is my turn, no it is your turn"... I am here sitting quiet and peaceful, patiently waiting for my turn.

Suddenly Ciccillo pops at the door, he looks at me and smiles.

I'm glad to see him again, his face is so familiar for me now.

How nice, he managed to have his shift changed to say hello to me and deal with my "treatment".

Remarkable!

The "machine" is different... but the process is always the same.

Besides him, there are two women doctors that peer at me, check my scar and draw strange marks on my skin with a golden phosphorescent liquid, a ritual, which looks like a rebus.

"During these days always take a lint with you, as this liquid could blot you, and it is indelible... so rub a lot of lotion, as your skin is peeling... we'll see you on Monday"...

Ok.

I don't know the reason but I walk away almost satisfied.

Outside the Sun welcomes me with all his warmth and this time it even warms up my heart.

I am in a good mood, despite everything.

The break had a good effect on me.

I took advantage to have a quick trip to Florence to visit maternal relatives. It's always very pleasant to meet all my cousins, after all, we grew up together and, when we were children, we lived the same experiences, so now, it only takes a glance to understand one another.

And then, I feel so beloved there.

My aunts always tell me particular episodes of my childhood, funny anecdotes that otherwise I couldn't remember, and every time they enable me to add a piece to my life's puzzle.

For them, you are always a little girl, they pamper you and make you really feel like that.

I love this.

"When you were a child, you were such a good girl, you were so beautiful and also so quiet, and silent"...

What a pity that, as we grow up, we waste ourselves.

27. *"Know-how" - Savoir Faire*

Now I realized what this program of "twenty-five + five" means. It is a bit like baste and then sew. An "had hoc" work, even better, controlled and guaranteed.

Doctors and radiation therapists are very professional and qualified people. They really must study everything besides medicine, chemistry, biology, anatomy, psycho ogy and so on.

Patients, very often, come here frightened, confused, and they try to make you feel at ease; they have that particular *"savoir faire"*, I never found, unfortunately, in the departments of any other hospital.

Or rather I found it only in pediatric departments, or at least, I hope so. To be a doctor, or a priest and a magistrate, should be a "mission"; as, by choosing this work, our lives, our souls and our destinies as well are in their hands. But they often forget this.

I got in touch, in spite of myself, with some doctors and judges because of my profession, anyway I missed the priests, as for them I hadn't the opportunity to widen my knowledge, the

latest contacts date back to my first communion and so many years have gone by since then. Sgrunt!

I couldn't give a definition about my relationship with God, but the fact that you write his name with a capital letter is already a sign of respect... it is an ambiguous relationship and, as I believe for many other people, it is made up a little "of convenience", that is to say:

"We search for Him and implore Him only in big difficulty moments, but then we forget Him". The thing is that I think having an absolute faith is a gift and, even if I am sorry about this, I am pretty sure that I do not possess it.

While I am getting undressed, I follow with my eyes every movement of the technicians that are craftily arranging, measuring, calibrating. They make me lie down in my new couch, in this diverse-blue room.
I am pleased to discover that, at least, here there is not that annoying stain on the ceiling, right there on the obliged trajectory of my gaze. I could just close my eyes to not see it.
Sometimes little things can bring us a great happiness.
Here everything is clearer, it would be almost perfect if there was also the magic of music. "It is not expected to be used" they answered, when I asked them about it.
What a pity!
I have always deeply felt its absence.

28. "My Father"

The sky is gray and it's raining, this year Spring is kind of weird. But although I am a bit meteoropathic, today the weather doesn't affect my mood or at least I try not to be affected. I'm trying to find the bright side and the selfish one of things too, since I can't go to the seaside yet.

My father accompanied me today, later we have lots of things to do together, with mom too, but he preferred to stay out and wait in his car. He can't absolutely enter an hospital, unless he is obliged to do it.

For this kind of support I surely cannot rely on him… for everything else, though, I must admit his absolute helpfulness. He is always ready to come and get me, to go to the Post Office, to the grocery, etc.. He is often smiling at others, especially in dance halls, and ready to help you in case of practical difficulties... From the outside a perfect father and husband as well. But I don't want to keep going at him, after all, he makes me feel a sense of protectiveness and, from my heart, I know that he loves me, and in his own way… he loves all his family.

As a child, I was his pride, because I was the only sporty one in my family and he would follow every competition of mine, especially during my athletic races, he would run by my side during the marathons, encouraging me and proudly telling everyone that I was his daughter.

He used to take me, enthusiastically to football matches, infusing me with the passion for our favourite team (maybe… it is the only interest that we have in common).

I truly know that he would have always preferred to have a son …but, after me, my sister was born.
However, that one was the only period in my life during which I felt my father's love and caring presence.

Ciccillo is sorry, as he can't look after me today.
I smile at him, "Don't worry, I have two other treatments after this, then who knows, I will come back and see you"… Even if I was pretty aware of the uncertainty of my assertion.
Instead of him there are a man and a woman, both of them just already seen but they look indifferents and they hastily carry out their duties quite mechanically, I think they are tired.
I ask them about some strange spots on my skin and, always mechanically, they reply "You simply need to rub a bit of alcohol, it will take a few days but eventually they will disappear". Only later I would discover, anyway, that alcohol is not very suitable in these cases, as your skin is burnt, so it could scald your skin even more.
"But who told you this bloody nonsense"… the lovable "Roman lady" exclaims, "You need to rub your skin gently with a cotton wad soaked in neutral cleansing milk".
Ok.

Outside it is hailing.
My father comes towards me carrying an umbrella, we look at each other… almost apologizing for our, now mutual, inability to love, or maybe only for the difficulty to show our emotions and address our love to each other.

29. "The Magic of Rome"

The large window is open and a ray of sunshine softly came in through touching my skin, I close my eyes, it is very pleasant.

Rome is like that!
One day is rainy and windy even in summer, but most of the times the Sun is the absolute protagonist of Roman seasons. It is largely for this reason, that I resolved to spend my life in this magic city.
Besides the noticeable fact that in Rome you can literally walk on history.
Every place, alley, *sanpietrino*[3], talks about Her. I often think about this, whenever I cover its ancient streets, the Imperial Forum, the *Appia Antica*, *Trastevere*, the heart of Rome, and especially by foot or by bicycle, you can really breathe its history.
Although it is, like all big metropolis, a chaotic city, with plenty of traffic and planning problems, here you can always find your "magic corner", an alley you did not remember to have covered, a monument, a church, a shiny fountain, a big statue, an almost living sculpture.
Works of art, masterpieces near at hand for all "gourmets" which leave you breathless.
Thank you Rome for being so beautifully unique!

---

[3] *Sanpietrini*, (also Sampietrini) is a typical kind of pavement as the habit of ancient Rome, usually situated in the heart of Rome and made up of small squared tiles of black porphyry, placed one next to the other.

"Come on, you are nearly done! Tomorrow it will be the last one, so you will, eventually, never see our ugly face again"…

The two technicians are cheerful today and pass on their good mood to me. All of them joke about my "hieroglyphics"

"Hey, in this period try not to "hit" on" a riddle solver, otherwise he will stop right there trying to solve the rebus"… then they burst out laughing and I did too after them.

Life is beautiful, despite everything, and full of wonderful nuances.

Before leaving I stop here in the garden and decide to sit on this sundrenched and inviting bench, a strong appeal that I can't ignore.

I start writing, enjoying the warmth of the sun, this light air which I deeply breath.

Summer is just around the corner.

"Hey beautiful, what are you writing, your memoirs"? he is the technician from before, who has gone out from the "bunker" as well, to breathe this Spring air.

"You know that, at least for this year, you can't sunbathe, don't you"?, with an almost reproaching tone.

Then, noticing my somewhat lost look, he smiles and reassures me:

"By the way, stay here, don't worry, these are not radiations that can harm you".

Ok.

And under the Sun I set out, slowly, with a big smile on my face and this delightful warmth on my skin.

30. "The Big Challenge"

My mother is here, again, dauntlessly by my side, keeping close.

She insisted to come but, nevertheless, she started this "adventure" with me and it is right to give her the chance to live the conclusion of this story.

Her look is always the same, with that veil of sadness mixed with resignation, but today with a glimmer of hope more.

She talks with the doctors, queries, inquires about everything, then she begs one of them to allow her to be there during my "treatment", since it is the last one, and she is too curious to see, with her own eyes, what they have been doing to her "little girl". "Please doctor, make me happy" and, fortunately, he agrees with a smile.

I always said that it takes little to be happy and also to make other people happy.

I look at her, she is so small but so vital... such a mom! The thought to have given her all this pain, against my will, really wrings my heart.

I will never stop thanking her for the love, strength and courage she gave me and, above all, for the way she faced these long and very dark months.

"It seems as an horror movie," I remember her exclaiming when she received the news, ... "Oh, it can't be true... why you?"

After all, everyone wonders the same.

Quite often you can hear "certain stories" on TV, but

you always listen to them quite absent-mindedly, as you are already accustomed to hear to all sorts of stories, as if it could never concern you, as if you could stay immune from it.

But when it happens to you, on the other hand, you feel so small, but so small, but at the same time so strong, but so strong ... a bit like a free climber who has to climb a mountain that gets higher and more insidious at every step, and when he finally hardly reaches the summit, he can taste the joy and the feeling of overcoming a big challenge, the challenge against the world... but on his own skin!

"Dulcis in Fundo" (Last but Not Least)

And as wisely said a genius of the cinema...

"In my next life I want to live backwards.
You start out dead and get that out of the way.
Then you wake up in an old people's home
feeling better every day.
You get kicked out for being too healthy,
go collect your pension, and then when
you start work, you get a gold watch
and a party of your first day.
You work for 40 years until you're young
enough to enjoy your retirement.
You party, drink alcohol, and are
generally promiscuous, then you
are ready for high school.
You then go to primary school,
you become a kid, you play.
you have no responsibilities,
you become a baby until you are born.
And then you spend your last 9 months floating in
luxurious spa like conditions with
central heating and room service
on tap, larger quarters every day
and then, Voilà!
You finish off as an orgasm!
I rest my case."

Brilliant!

List of Literary Awards

"Just a Skin Matter" (*É questione di pelle*) winner of the First **"Narra il Saggio"** (*Tell the Essay)* Literary Prize for unpublished narrative works, 2008, Miele Publisher; Gagliano del Capo (Lecce).

Winner of the only placement for long stories of the Fifth **"Le Donne raccontano"** (*Women tell*) Literary Prize, 2008/2009, WomanEurope (EuropaDonna); Pontedera

Finalist at the Third "ALBEROANDRONICO" Literary Prize for published works, 2010 Campidoglio - Rome;

Semifinalist at the Sixteenth Literary Prize "Author's Pen Award" (*Trofeo Penna d'Autore*) for published works, 2010 Torino.

Finalist at the first Literary Prize "**A Memoria di Donna**". 2010, Agropoli (SA)

Finalist at the first Literary Prize **"La Forza dei sentimenti"**, 2010, Rome.

Gabriella Franceschini was born on 5 October 1961, in Tripoli, Libya, of both Sicilian and Umbrian origins, but she has lived in Rome for great part of her existence. At the moment she is a clerk. She has always had a keen interest in photography and adventure. She also travelled extensively...as she herself says: "I am always looking for my own place in the world."

"Just a skin matter" is her first work.

CONTENTS

Lightning Source UK Ltd.
Milton Keynes UK
UKOW051509071011

179934UK00001B/20/P